About the NCCN Guidelines for Patients®

National Comprehensive Cancer Network®

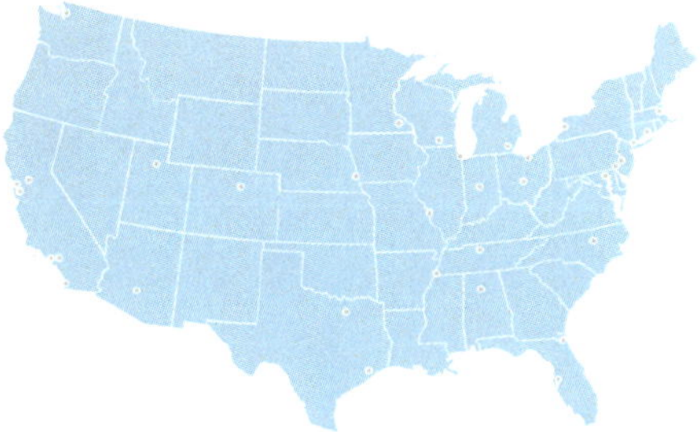

Did you know that top cancer centers across the United States work together to improve cancer care? This alliance of leading cancer centers is called the National Comprehensive Cancer Network® (NCCN®).

Cancer care is always changing. NCCN develops evidence-based cancer care recommendations used by health care providers worldwide. These frequently updated recommendations are the NCCN Clinical Practice Guidelines in Oncology (NCCN Guidelines®). The NCCN Guidelines for Patients plainly explain these expert recommendations for people with cancer and caregivers.

These NCCN Guidelines for Patients are based on the NCCN Clinical Practice Guidelines in Oncology (NCCN Guidelines®) for Myelodysplastic Syndromes, Version 3.2024 – July 25, 2024.

View the NCCN Guidelines for Patients free online
NCCN.org/patientguidelines

Find an NCCN Cancer Center near you
NCCN.org/cancercenters

Connect with us

Supporters

NATIONAL COMPREHENSIVE CANCER NETWORK® NCCN FOUNDATION
Guiding Treatment. Changing Lives.

NCCN Guidelines for Patients are supported by funding from the NCCN Foundation®

NCCN Foundation gratefully acknowledges the following corporate supporters for helping to make available these NCCN Guidelines for Patients: AbbVie, Bristol Myers Squibb, Servier, and Taiho Oncology, Inc.

NCCN independently adapts, updates, and hosts the NCCN Guidelines for Patients. Our corporate supporters do not participate in the development of the NCCN Guidelines for Patients and are not responsible for the content and recommendations contained therein.

To make a gift or learn more, visit online or email

NCCNFoundation.org/donate

PatientGuidelines@NCCN.org

Contents

NCCN Foundation seeks to support the millions of patients and their families affected by a cancer diagnosis by funding and distributing NCCN Guidelines for Patients. NCCN Foundation is also committed to advancing cancer treatment by funding the nation's promising doctors at the center of innovation in cancer research. For more details and the full library of patient and caregiver resources, visit NCCN.org/patients.

National Comprehensive Cancer Network (NCCN) and NCCN Foundation
3025 Chemical Road, Suite 100, Plymouth Meeting, PA 19462 USA

1
What is MDS?

Myelodysplastic syndromes (MDS) are a group of rare bone marrow disorders and are considered to be a form of blood cancer. In MDS, the bone marrow doesn't make enough healthy blood cells, which can cause low blood cell counts. This chapter explains MDS.

Myelodysplastic syndromes (MDS) are a group of rare bone marrow disorders.

- **myelo-** means "bone marrow"

Your bone marrow is the soft material inside your bones where blood cells are made.

- **dysplastic** means "abnormal development"

Put together, myelodysplastic syndromes are diseases where the bone marrow fails to produce normal blood cells correctly.

Is MDS considered cancer?

MDS is a type of cancer. Cancer occurs when cells don't function as intended and begin growing out of control.

In MDS, the cells in the bone marrow become abnormal. These abnormal cells crowd out normal blood cells.

In healthy bone marrow, undeveloped cells called stem cells (which look immature in the bone marrow and are called "blasts") develop into the blood cells necessary for healthy living.

In normal healthy bone marrow, blasts make up about 1 percent (1%) to 2 percent (2%) of all blood cells and act as seeds for the growth of all normal types of cells. After they fully develop in the bone marrow, new blood cells leave the bone marrow and enter the peripheral blood to perform their assigned jobs:

- Red blood cells: Transport oxygen throughout the body
- White blood cells: Fight infection
- Platelets: Form blood clots in response to injury

However, in MDS, stem cells in the bone marrow develop genetic errors that affect their ability to grow. Cells that are produced by these damaged stem cells do not grow normally.

They remain relatively immature when looking under the microscope and often fail to develop into adult cells. These "dysplastic" (abnormal) cells take up space and nutrients in the bone marrow. As a result, they outgrow the healthy cells and make it harder for normal cells to develop.

MDS may get worse over time. In some cases, it may develop into a faster-growing cancer called acute myeloid leukemia (AML). This occurs when more and more abnormal cells build up and fill up the bone marrow space like weeds in a garden.

A person is considered to have AML if they have a blast percentage of 20 percent (20%), but experts have been considering lowering this number to 10 percent (10%).

About 1 out of 3 people with MDS, who have other risk factors, may develop AML. For more information, read the *NCCN Guidelines for Patients: Acute Myeloid Leukemia*, available at NCCN.org/patientguidelines and on the Patient Guides for Cancer app.

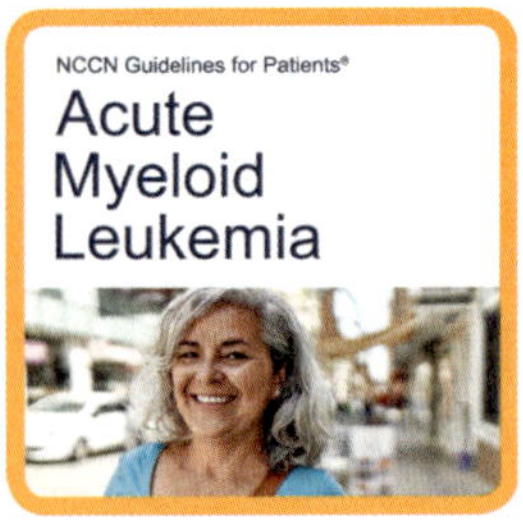

Read on to learn more about the risk factors for MDS.

Risk factors for MDS

Risk factors don't necessarily cause cancer. But having risk factors can increase the chances of getting cancer. Risk factors for MDS include:

- Older age: The average person with MDS is in their 70s or 80s
- Sex: MDS is more common in people assigned male at birth than those assigned female
- Previous cancer treatment: Chemotherapy and radiation therapy
- Inherited genetic syndromes: Including Fanconi anemia, Shwachman-Diamond syndrome, telomere biology disorders, and others
- Having a relative with MDS: Passed through generations of a family due to a known gene mutation
- Smoking
- Exposure to benzene

How severe is MDS?

You may be wondering how severe MDS can be. The answer to this question is that it depends entirely on the person. Some people won't have symptoms or need treatment for years, while others will need aggressive treatment for their symptoms right away.

On the other hand, many patients fall between these two extremes and may need treatment occasionally for symptoms that come and go.

Finally, as you'll see throughout this book, there is also a risk of MDS transforming into a serious form of leukemia – AML. It's a fast-growing form of leukemia and can be challenging to treat.

In Chapter 2, we'll discuss the categories used for levels of MDS risk. You can calculate your level of risk with your care team or use a calculator online, which can help guide your treatment decisions.

Symptoms of MDS

MDS causes low levels of one or more types of blood cells. This shortage is called a cytopenia. Specific cytopenias have different names:

- Anemia is a lack of healthy red blood cells.
- Leukopenia is a lack of white blood cells.
- Thrombocytopenia is a lack of healthy platelets.

Anemia

Anemia is often the first cytopenia recognized in a person with MDS. This means you have a lower-than-normal red blood cell count. You may experience the following if you have anemia:

- Feel sleepy or tiredness that doesn't get better with rest
- Loss of appetite
- Pale skin
- Chest pain
- Shortness of breath
- Irregular or rapid heartbeat
- Cold hands and feet

Blood cell formation

Bone marrow contains stem cells. A blood stem cell is an immature cell that can develop into a red blood cell, white blood cell, or platelet.

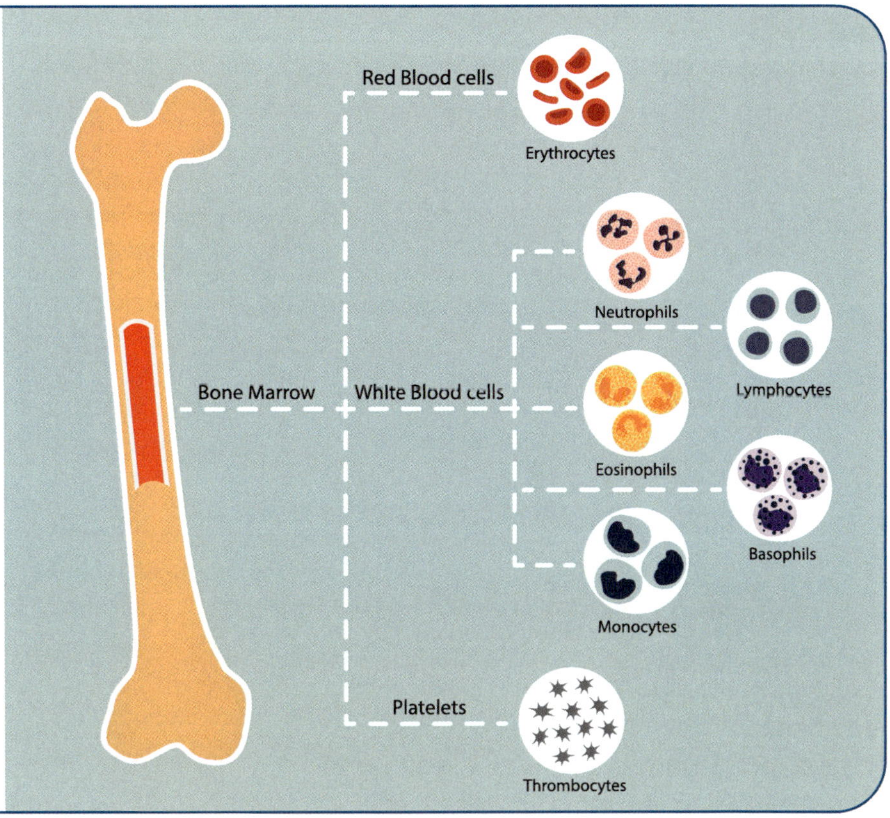

Leukopenia

Leukopenia is a drop in white blood cells. A shortage of white blood cells means there are fewer disease-fighting cells (leukocytes) in your blood.

Symptoms of leukopenia include:

- Fever
- Swelling and redness (inflammation) in and around the mouth
- Frequent infections
- Infections that don't go away

Neutropenia

Neutropenia (a type of leukopenia) refers to a decrease in neutrophils, the most common type of white blood cell. A lack of neutrophils can lead to frequent or severe infections.

A person with neutropenia may experience:

- Frequent fevers or infections
- Bladder infections that are painful or make you urinate more often
- Lung infections that cause coughing and difficulty breathing
- Mouth sores
- Sinus infections
- Skin infections

Thrombocytopenia

Platelets help control bleeding and heal wounds by forming blood clots. When you have a shortage of healthy platelets, that's called thrombocytopenia. In rare cases, the number of platelets drops so low that blood won't clot, and you can start bleeding internally.

Bleeding that will not stop is considered a medical emergency. If you have bleeding that will not stop, go to the emergency room or call 911.

If you have a low platelet count, you may experience:

- Unexplained bruising or bleeding
- Nose bleeds
- Bleeding gums, especially after brushing your teeth
- Tiny, flat red spots under your skin (petechiae)
- Heavier than normal menstrual periods

Can MDS be cured?

A bone marrow transplant can be a cure for some types of MDS. This treatment requires good underlying health and organ function to tolerate the side effects.

While not everyone can be cured, anyone with MDS can receive treatment to reduce symptoms and prolong life. Some people don't require treatment for years, while others need treatment, such as chemotherapy or immunotherapy, right away.

Some types of MDS also come with a greater risk of developing AML.

Don't forget: there are always treatment options. Talk with your care team to decide what treatment is best for you.

Key points

- Myelodysplastic syndromes (MDS) are a group of cancers that affect blood cells in the bone marrow and bloodstream.
- In MDS, the bone marrow makes abnormal blood cells and doesn't make enough healthy, mature blood cells for the body.
- When you have low count of a type of blood cell, it's called cytopenia.
- Anemia is a low red blood cell count and, when unexplained, is usually the first sign of MDS.
- MDS is divided into types based on the features of the bone marrow and blood cells, and genetic abnormalities.
- MDS can sometimes be cured with a stem cell transplant in certain people. Everyone with MDS can be treated to slow the disease and reduce symptoms.

2
Testing for MDS

Testing is needed to diagnose and treat myelodysplastic syndromes (MDS). This chapter presents an overview of required tests and those you might receive.

Your provider needs to run tests to properly diagnose and treat myelodysplastic syndromes (MDS). Some of those tests involve taking some of your blood from a vein or your bone marrow; others might involve answering a few questions about your health.

More tests may involve checking your body for signs of disease. Those tests are detailed in this chapter.

Medical history

A medical history is a record of all health issues and treatments you've had in your life. Be prepared to list any illness or injury and when it happened.

- Bring a list of any medicines you take, including over-the-counter medicines, herbs, or supplements.
- A medical history helps determine which treatment option is best for you.

Family history

Some cancers and other diseases can run in families. Your health care provider will ask about the health history of family members who are blood relatives. This information is called a family history.

Before you visit with your health care provider, you may want to ask your biological family members about their health issues like heart disease, cancer, and diabetes and what age they were diagnosed.

Documentation of transfusion

Bring any information you may have on your previous transfusions. This will be helpful for your health care provider in developing your treatment plan.

Be ready to tell your doctor about your medical history, including any family history of cancer.

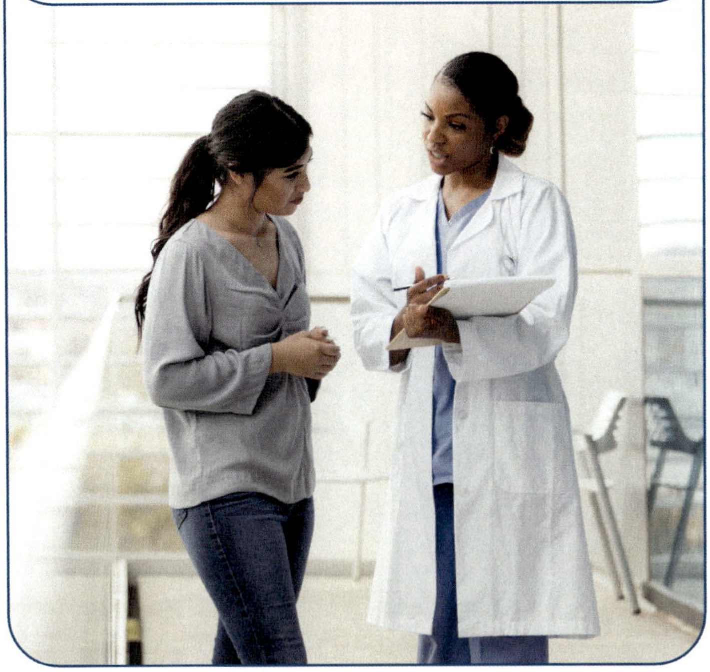

Physical exam

A physical exam checks your body for signs of disease.

A health care provider may:

- Check your temperature, blood pressure, pulse, and breathing rate
- Check your weight
- Listen to your lungs and heart
- Look in your eyes, ears, nose, and throat
- Feel and apply pressure to parts of your body to see if organs are of normal size, are soft or hard, or cause pain when touched

A list of necessary and optional testing can be found in **Guide 1.**

Guide 1
Tests for MDS

	• Medical history and physical exam • Documentation of transfusion history
Needed or recommended	• Complete blood count (CBC), platelets, differential, reticulocyte count • Examination of peripheral blood smear • Bone marrow aspiration with iron stain and for molecular/myeloid mutation panel and standard chromosome/karyotyping studies • Serum erythropoietin (EPO) (prior to red blood cell [RBC] transfusion) • RBC folate, vitamin B12 evaluation • Serum ferritin, iron, total iron-binding capacity (TIBC) • Thyroid-stimulating hormone (TSH) • Lactate dehydrogenase (LDH) • Genetic testing for somatic mutations (acquired mutations) • Molecular and genetic testing for hereditary hematologic malignancy predisposition (mainly for patients under age 50 years) • HIV testing • Bone marrow sample for fibrosis
Optional (if needed)	Evaluation of copper deficiency
	Distinction from congenital sideroblastic anemia (CSA)

Blood tests

Blood tests check for signs of disease and how well organs are working. They require a blood sample, which is removed through a needle placed into your vein.

The blood sample will then be sent to a lab for testing. At the lab, a pathologist (an expert in lab medicine) will examine the blood sample with a microscope and perform other tests outlined below.

Complete blood count

A complete blood count (CBC) measures the levels of red blood cells (RBCs), white blood cells (WBCs), and platelets in your blood. A CBC looks for many illnesses, including anemia, infections, and leukemia.

Anemia symptoms and testing

Symptoms depend on your specific type of anemia. Minor symptoms can be so mild that they go unnoticed. As the body loses more iron and anemia gets worse, symptoms also get worse.

If you have symptoms of anemia, your health care provider will perform a series of tests to identify the type of anemia and how severe it is. For a full list of tests for all cytopenias, **see Guide 2.**

Differential

A differential counts the number of each type of WBC. There are 5 types of WBCs: neutrophils, lymphocytes, monocytes, eosinophils, and basophils.

A differential also checks if the WBC counts are in balance with each other. Your health care provider may be able to determine the cause of an abnormal WBC count from this test.

Guide 2 **Testing for cytopenias**
Physical exam
Complete blood count (CBC), platelets, differential, reticulocyte count
Examination of peripheral blood smear
Bone marrow aspiration with iron stain, biopsy, and cytogenetics
Serum erythropoietin (EPO) level

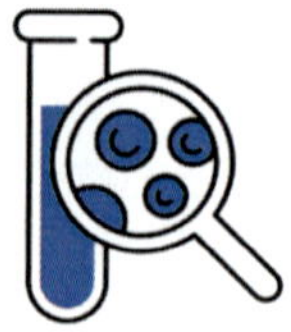

Types of anemia

Anemia associated with bone marrow disease

Anemia associated with bone marrow disease affects the blood produced in your bone marrow. This anemia includes a variety of diseases, such as leukemia, MDS, and myelofibrosis.

Aplastic anemia

In aplastic anemia, normal blood cell production slows or stops. This occurs because bone marrow stem cells are damaged. The number of stem cells also goes down because they cannot replicate themselves or are being destroyed by a part of the immune system.

Hemolytic anemia

Hemolytic anemia occurs when red blood cells are destroyed faster than bone marrow can replace them. Hemolytic anemia can be acquired in two ways: you can inherit it or develop it later in life.

Iron deficiency anemia

Iron deficiency anemia is the most common type of anemia. It is caused by a lack of iron in your body. Your bone marrow needs iron to make hemoglobin. Hemoglobin is needed to transport oxygen throughout the body from your lungs. Without enough iron, your body can't produce enough hemoglobin for red blood cells.

Sickle cell anemia

Sickle cell anemia is an inherited and serious condition. It is caused by a defective form of hemoglobin that forces red blood cells to take on an abnormal crescent moon (sickle) shape. The irregular blood cells die too soon, resulting in an ongoing shortage of red blood cells.

Vitamin deficiency anemia

Vitamins (specifically folate, vitamin B12, and vitamin C) are essential to make healthy red blood cells. Vitamin deficiency anemia can occur if you do not eat enough foods that have folate, vitamin B12, or vitamin C. It can also occur if your body has trouble absorbing or processing these vitamins.

Reticulocyte count

Reticulocytes are immature red blood cells that are produced in your bone marrow and released into the peripheral blood (bone marrow blood). A reticulocyte count can help your health care provider learn if your bone marrow is able to produce red blood cells in response to the development of anemia.

This test may also help your health care provider find out the cause of anemia. The body's normal response to anemia is for the bone marrow to make more reticulocytes. A low reticulocyte count is a sign that the bone marrow isn't working to produce more red blood cells.

Blood smear

In a blood smear test, a drop of blood is placed on a slide so it can be viewed with a microscope. A pathologist will look at cell size, shape, type, and maturity. This test is also used to count the different types of blood cells, which helps to determine if blood cells are abnormal in shape or size (dysplasia).

A blood smear test may also be used to check for blast cells in the bloodstream. Blast cells are normally found in the bone marrow, but in some cases of MDS, blast cells may be found in the bloodstream.

Serum erythropoietin

Erythropoietin (EPO) helps to stimulate bone marrow to make more red blood cells. The body makes EPO when it detects a low level of oxygen in red blood cells.

By measuring the amount of EPO in the blood, your health care provider may be able to figure out the cause of anemia. People with anemia from MDS typically have an EPO level that is higher than normal.

Iron, ferritin, folate, and vitamin B12

Iron is considered essential because it is needed to make hemoglobin. Hemoglobin is the protein in red blood cells that carries oxygen. Ferritin is a protein in your blood that contains iron.

A ferritin test will help your provider understand how much iron is in your body. If the blood ferritin test is lower than normal, it indicates an iron deficiency. As a result, you could be anemic. If the ferritin test is higher than normal, it could indicate you are storing too much iron.

Folate and vitamin B12 are nutrients in the body that are needed to make red blood cells. A shortage of folate or B12 can cause anemia.

Thyroid-stimulating hormone

Your thyroid makes hormones to control how fast your body uses energy. Your health care provider will test the amount of thyroid-stimulating hormone (TSH) in your blood. A high level of TSH in your blood is a sign that your thyroid is not making enough hormones. If your thyroid does not make enough hormones, it can lead to anemia.

Copper level

Copper is a mineral that helps with many processes in the body. A low level of copper can cause the number of red blood cells and white blood cells to be low. It can also cause blood cells to have an abnormal size or shape.

While not a standard test for MDS,testing for copper level may be done in certain cases to rule out other causes of the abnormal appearance or number of blood cells.

HIV testing

Human immunodeficiency virus (HIV) can cause low blood cell counts. It can also cause blood cells to have an abnormal size or shape. In certain cases, tests may be done to rule out HIV as the cause of these symptoms.

HLA typing

A human leukocyte antigen (HLA) is a protein found on the surface of most cells. It plays an important role in your body's immune response. HLA typing is a test that detects a person's HLA type.

HLAs are unique to each person. They mark your body's cells. Your body detects these markers to tell which cells are yours. All your cells have the same set of HLAs. Each person's set of HLAs is called the HLA type or tissue type.

This test is required before a donor blood stem cell transplant, so it's performed early on. Your proteins will be compared to the donor's white blood cells to see how many proteins are the same to find the best match. This can take some time.

If it's not the best match possible, your body will reject the donor cells, or the donor cells will react against your body. Blood samples from you and your blood relatives will be tested first.

Flow cytometry

Flow cytometry involves adding a light-sensitive dye to cells. The cells are passed through a beam of light in a machine. The machine measures the number, size, shape, and proteins found on the surface of thousands of cells.

In some cases of MDS, this test may be used to identify the specific type of cells present.

Blood tests are the main method used to determine the best course of treatment.

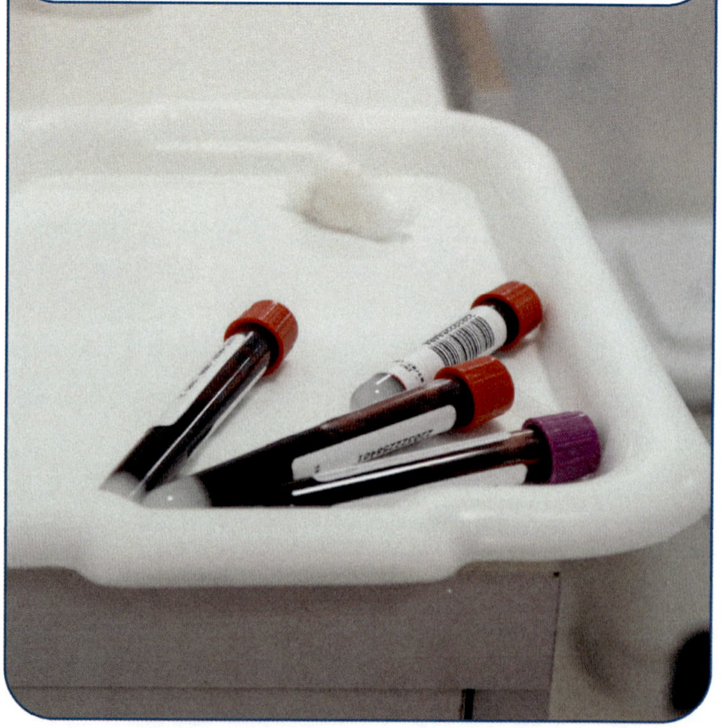

Bone marrow tests

Bone marrow is tested to diagnose and classify the type of MDS. This test may also be repeated to tell if the MDS is responding to treatment or is transforming into acute myeloid leukemia (AML).

Two types of bone marrow tests are often done at the same time:

- Aspiration
- Biopsy

A bone marrow aspiration takes some of the liquid out of the spongy tissue of the marrow. A biopsy takes a piece of the marrow. For aspiration, a hollow needle will be pushed through your skin and into the bone. Liquid bone marrow will then be drawn into a syringe.

For the biopsy, a needle will be used to remove a core sample of bone with marrow. The samples will be sent to a lab for testing. You may feel bone pain in your hip for a few days. Your skin may bruise.

The samples are usually taken from the back of the hip bone (pelvis). Ask your provider about the type of bone marrow test you might have, where the sample will be taken, and if you will be given a medicine to help you relax.

Removing bone marrow samples

Samples of your bone marrow may need to be removed and tested for diagnosis or treatment planning. A bone marrow aspiration removes a small amount of liquid bone marrow. A bone marrow biopsy removes a small piece of bone with marrow. These procedures are often done on the back of the hip one after the other.

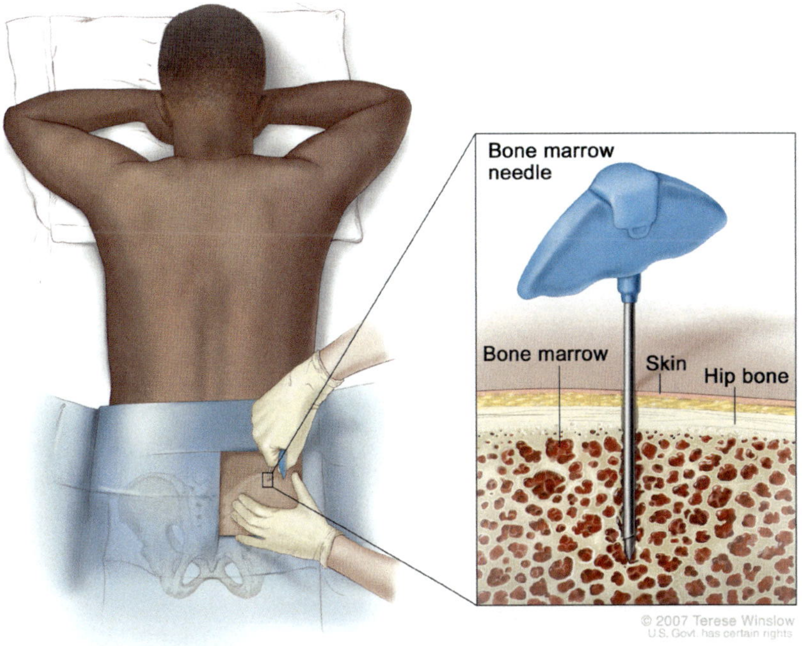

Genetic tests

If you are suspected of having MDS, you may receive tests to look for evidence of a cancer predisposition syndrome that is inherited in your family line. Some patients who develop MDS have been born with a mutation that is present in every cell in their body ("a germline mutation").

People who have germline mutations can be at risk for different types of cancer, not just MDS, and might have specific physical findings such as early hair graying or specific skin or bone findings.

Your doctor will ask you about your personal and family history of cancer as well as whether you yourself have had more than one type of cancer. If you have more than two immediate relatives with cancer or have a diagnosis of two or more cancers, this increases the chance that you might have a cancer predisposition syndrome. Germline genetic testing can be done on samples from any tissue of your body (blood, skin, hair, spit).

Specific testing to evaluate the diagnosis of MDS requires samples obtained from bone marrow aspirations or biopsies.

Inside our cells are DNA molecules. These molecules are tightly packaged into what is called a chromosome.

Chromosomes contain most of the genetic information in a cell. Most human cells contain 23 pairs of chromosomes for a total of 46 chromosomes.

Each chromosome contains thousands of genes. Genes tell cells what to do and what to become.

The following are some genetic tests that may be done.

Cytogenetic testing

Cytogenetic testing is the study of chromosomes. Samples of tissue, blood, or bone marrow are tested to look for changes or defects in chromosomes.

There are many types of chromosome defects. Part of a chromosome, or a whole chromosome, may be missing. Or there may be an extra copy of a chromosome.

Health care providers use symbols and shortened terms to describe the different types of chromosome changes. A missing chromosome or missing part of a chromosome is noted by a minus sign (-) or the word "del" for deletion. An extra copy of a chromosome is noted by a plus sign (+).

Examples of chromosome defects in MDS include:

- del(5q) and 5q- both mean that the "q" or longer part of chromosome 5 is missing
- -7 and del(7) both mean that a copy of chromosome 7 is missing
- +7 means that there is an extra copy of chromosome 7

Half of people with MDS have abnormal chromosomes. The most common abnormalities in MDS are found on chromosomes 5, 7, 8, and 20.

Identifying the type and number of chromosome changes helps health care providers assess the likely outcome (prognosis) for your MDS. This information can also help guide treatment options.

FISH

Fluorescence in situ hybridization (FISH) is a test that identifies the genetic material in a person's cells. FISH testing can be done on samples of blood or bone marrow. This test detects specific gene or chromosome changes that are common and known to affect patients with MDS.

Karyotype

A karyotype is a genetic test that produces an image of a person's chromosomes. The test is used to look for abnormal numbers or structures of chromosomes.

Molecular testing

Molecular testing is used to find small changes in genes. It is more sensitive than either karyotype or FISH. Molecular testing is done on a sample of blood or bone marrow removed from your body.

DNA sequencing

More than 50 different gene mutations have been repeatedly found in people with MDS. These are called recurrent gene mutations. DNA sequencing is a test that can identify mistakes within genes.

Health care providers use this test to find out which recurrent gene mutations are present in MDS cells. Certain mutations are linked with a better or worse prognosis or can help predict response to different treatments. Health care providers may test for these common mutations to help plan treatment.

What are the types of MDS?

MDS is broken up into types based on bone marrow and blood cell features as well as certain genetic abnormalities.

The World Health Organization (WHO) separates MDS into groups based on genetic mutations (changes in your DNA) you may have or how the cells within the bone marrow look under a microscope. This includes these specific factors:

- How many blood cells in the bone marrow look abnormal (known as dysplasia)
- How many types of low blood cell counts are found (known as cytopenia)
- How many very early forms of blood cells (blasts) are in the bone marrow or bloodstream
    - The more blasts found in the bloodstream, the worse the MDS can be
- Certain chromosome and genetic changes in the bone marrow cells

Based on these factors, the WHO system recognizes 7 main types of MDS. They are described next.

For more information on types of MDS, **see Guide 3.**

MDS types grouped by genetics

MDS with low blasts and isolated 5q deletion (MDS-5q)

Someone with MDS with low blasts and isolated 5q deletion has at least one abnormal chromosome change in their cells in the bone marrow. This change is called 5q, which means that part of chromosome 5 is missing (deleted). In some circumstances, one additional abnormal chromosome may also be present.

"Low blasts" means that less than 5 percent (5%) of cells in the bone marrow are blast cells (immature blood cells) and less than 2 percent (2%) of cells in the peripheral blood (blood in the bone) are blast cells.

Guide 3
Types of MDS

MDS	MDS with low blasts and isolated 5q deletion (MDS-5q) MDS with low blasts and *SF3B1* mutation (MDS-*SF3B1*) MDS with biallelic *TP53* inactivation (MDS-bi*TP53*) MDS with low blasts (MDS-LB) MDS, hypoplastic (MDS-h) MDS with increased blasts 1 (MDS-IB1) MDS with increased blasts 2 (MDS-IB2) MDS with fibrosis (MDS-f)
MDS/MPN overlap syndromes	CMML-1 CMML-2 MDS/MPN with neutrophilia MDS/MPN with *mSF3B1* and thrombocytosis MDS/MPN, not otherwise specified (NOS)
Acute myeloid leukemia (AML)	See *NCCN Guidelines for Patients: Acute Myeloid Leukemia*

The 5q deletion affects the production of red blood cells. As a result, people with this mutation tend to have anemia. 5q deletion accounts for 15 percent of MDS cases and tends to be more common in older people assigned female at birth than those assigned male. People with this type of MDS can live a long life and rarely develop AML.

MDS with low blasts and *SF3B1* mutation (MDS-*SF3B1*)
Someone with MDS with low blasts and *SF3B1* mutation has a mutation in the *SF3B1* gene. Typically, they carry no other existing mutations. This type was originally called MDS with ring sideroblasts (MDS-RS) or refractory anemia with ring sideroblasts (RARS).

MDS-*SF3B1* is described as red blood cells containing rings of iron deposits (ring sideroblasts). These ring sideroblasts are leftovers of improper cell development.

This type most often affects older people or people of late middle age. There is a low risk of developing AML.

"Low blasts" means that less than 5 percent of cells in the bone marrow are blast cells (immature blood cells) and less than 2 percent of cells in the peripheral blood (blood in the bone) are blast cells.

MDS with biallelic *TP53* inactivation (MDS-biTP53)
Someone with MDS with biallelic *TP53* inactivation has a mutation in both copies of the *TP53* gene, which is responsible for controlling the process of cell death. For most cancers like MDS, *TP53* is necessary for getting rid of abnormal cells.

Most people have two copies of every gene in their chromosomes, with some exceptions —one from each parent. When *TP53* is inactivated in both copies, this is considered a "biallelic" inactivation.

The blast cell count tends to be higher for MDS-bi*TP53*, meaning 20 percent or less of cells in the bone marrow and the peripheral blood are blast cells.

About 1 in 10 people with MDS have *TP53* inactivation. Of these, 2 in 3 have biallelic *TP53* inactivation. Prognosis (outcome) is worse than in the other genetic types of MDS.

MDS with biallelic *TP53* inactivation can quickly turn into AML.

MDS types grouped by what the cells look like

MDS with low blasts (MDS-LB)
Someone with MDS with low blasts means that less than 5 percent of cells in the bone marrow are blast cells (immature blood cells) and less than 2 percent of cells in the peripheral blood (blood in the bone) are blasts. This is the most common type of MDS.

This type was originally called MDS with single lineage dysplasia, or MDS with multilineage dysplasia, depending on the symptoms. Some providers may still use these terms but they're considered optional today.

Some people with MDS with low blasts have 1 or more cytopenias (one or more blood cell types are lower than they should be) and abnormal cells in the bone marrow (dysplasias).

Blood and bone marrow are always involved. At least 2 types of blood counts are low and have an abnormal appearance under a microscope (dysplasia). This type of MDS includes childhood MDS, though it is very rare.

MDS, hypoplastic (MDS-h)
Someone with hypoplastic MDS has less than approximately 25 percent bone marrow cellularity, depending on their age. This means that there are fewer blood cells in the bone marrow. This is caused by unhealthy T-cells attacking healthy stem cells, lowering the pool of cells in the bone marrow as a result.

Hypoplastic MDS accounts for 10 to 15 percent of all MDS diagnoses. They tend to not respond well to chemotherapy treatments, but they can be more likely to respond to treatments used for aplastic anemia.

The rate of progression of MDS-h into AML is low.

MDS with increased blasts (MDS-IB1 + MDS-IB2)
A person with MDS with increased blasts has more immature blood cells than normal in the bone marrow.

This type of MDS is broken up into two types based on the number of increased blasts (MDS-IB1 and MDS-IB2). Those with MDS-IB1 have 5 to 9 percent of blasts in the bone marrow and 2 to 4 percent in the peripheral blood. Those with MDS-IB2 have 10 to 19 percent of blasts in the bone marrow and 5 to 19 percent in the peripheral blood.

It is one of the types of MDS most likely to turn into AML, with the risk being higher for MDS-IB2 than for MDS-IB1.

This type was originally called MDS with excess blasts 1 and 2 (MDS-EB1 + MDS-EB2).

MDS with fibrosis (MDS-f)
Someone with MDS with fibrosis (MDS-f) has 5 to 19 percent of blasts in the bone marrow, and 2 to 19 percent of blasts in the peripheral blood. This is considered a subtype of MDS with increased blasts. There also is fibrosis (scarring) in the bone marrow, typically called myelofibrosis.

Myelofibrosis can cause symptoms such as:

- Fatigue
- Shortness of breath
- Bleeding and bruising
- Abdominal pain
- Itchy skin
- Unexplained fever
- Unexplained weight loss

People with this subtype of MDS tend to have multiple cytopenias and survival rates aren't favorable.

For more information on myelofibrosis, read the *NCCN Guidelines for Patients: Myeloproliferative Neoplasms,* available at NCCN.org/patientguidelines and on the Patient Guides for Cancer app.

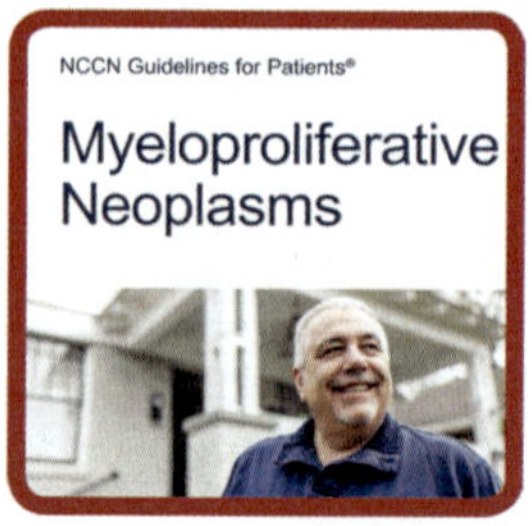

Scoring and risk groups

MDS severity is rated through a scoring system. The score is used to determine the likely outcome (prognosis) of MDS and to help develop a treatment plan. A rating, called a risk score, is used to classify MDS into risk groups.

This section describes the key factors and scoring systems used to determine MDS severity.

Prognostic factors

Prognosis is a prediction of the pattern and outcome of a disease. MDS treatment planning includes an assessment of the outcome for MDS. A key aspect of the outcome of MDS is the chance that it will turn into AML.

Certain factors related to your blood counts, bone marrow assessment, and karyotype/molecular profile affect the outcome of MDS. These are called prognostic factors.

These factors will be used to help decide if cancer treatment is needed right away and how intensive treatment needs to be.

These factors include:

- The MDS subtype
- The number and severity of low blood cell counts (cytopenias)
- The percent of blast cells in the bone marrow
- The type and number of chromosome changes
- The type and number of mutations identified by gene sequencing

Some factors are linked with better outcomes or a lower chance that MDS will turn into AML. Other factors help to predict the response to treatment.

Based on these prognostic factors, a scoring system is used to rate and classify the severity of MDS. This score can be calculated by your care team.

There are also calculators online that can use data from your recent test results, but discuss these with your care team before you take them seriously.

If your numbers add up to a lower score, you have a lower risk of MDS becoming AML. However, if your score is higher, you have a higher risk of MDS becoming AML.

There are three main prognostic scoring systems for MDS:

- IPSS-R (Revised International Prognostic Scoring System)
- WPSS (WHO classification-based Prognostic Scoring System)
- IPSS-M (International Prognostic Scoring System Molecular)

Each scoring system is described next.

IPSS-R

Most treatment providers and the NCCN Guidelines use the IPSS-R for their treatment recommendations.

The IPSS-R is different because it scores the types and severity of low blood cell counts.

It also scores a wider range of chromosome changes.

IPSS-R classifies MDS into 5 risk groups:

- Very low risk
- Low risk
- Intermediate risk
- High risk
- Very high risk

These 5 risk groups are divided into two basic risk categories: lower-risk MDS and higher-risk MDS.

The "lower-risk" MDS group includes anyone with a very low, low, or intermediate risk of disease.

"Higher-risk" MDS includes those with an intermediate, high, or very high risk of disease.

WPSS

The WPSS is not used as often as the IPSS-R. WPSS differs from the other systems because it includes the MDS subtype as a prognostic factor. As for low blood cell counts, the WPSS gives a score based on the presence or absence of severe anemia.

IPSS-M

The IPSS-M is a scoring system that takes into account blood counts, blast percentage, IPSS-R risk categories, genetics, and molecular sequencing results and provides time estimates for survival and AML transformation.

IPSS-M classifies MDS into 6 risk groups:

- Very low
- Low
- Moderate low
- Moderate high
- High
- Very high

The MDS Foundation has an IPSS-M calculator available on its website, available at: https://www.mds-foundation.org/additional-tools. Discuss the results with your care team.

The "lower-risk" MDS group includes anyone with a very low, low, or moderate-low risk of disease.

"Higher-risk" MDS includes those with a moderate-high, high, or very high risk of disease.

These scoring systems and risk groups do not predict how MDS will respond to treatment. They only help predict how MDS may behave over time without treatment.

Second opinions

It's normal to want to start treatment as soon as possible. While MDS should not be ignored, there is usually time to have another care provider review your test results and suggest a treatment plan.

For rare cancers like MDS, you should always have a second opinion to confirm your diagnosis and determine the best treatment goals for you.

Things you can do to prepare:

- Check with your insurance company about its rules on second opinions. There may be out-of-pocket costs to see health care providers who are not part of your insurance plan.
- Make plans to have copies of all your records sent to the health care provider you will see for your second opinion.
- Search for MDS providers or use the MDS Foundation's list of MDS care centers to get you started.

Key points

- A medical history, physical exam, and blood tests can reveal signs of cancer.
- A variety of blood tests are done to assess the extent and cause of low blood cell counts.
- Bone marrow tests are used to assess the prognosis of myelodysplastic syndromes (MDS). A bone marrow biopsy removes a piece of bone and marrow to test for cancer cells.
- A bone marrow aspiration removes liquid marrow.
- Genetic tests check for abnormal changes (mutations) in the genes and chromosomes of MDS cells. It is common for MDS cells to have genetic mutations.
- A risk score is a rating of the severity of MDS. It describes how slow or fast MDS will likely progress without treatment.
- When planning treatment, health care providers look at the risk groups in terms of "lower-risk" MDS and "higher-risk" MDS.

3
Treating MDS

There is more than one treatment for myelodysplastic syndromes (MDS). This chapter talks about the types of treatment and what to expect. Not everyone will receive the same treatment. Work with your care team to determine the best treatment option for your type of MDS.

There are several treatment possibilities for myelodysplastic syndromes (MDS):

- Chemotherapy
- Immunotherapy
- Erythroid maturation agents
- Immunomodulators
- Hematopoietic cell transplant (HCT) (bone marrow transplant)
- Enrolling in a clinical trial (this is a preferred treatment for MDS)

This chapter explains all these treatment possibilities and how they work. There's also information about clinical trials and supportive care. Discuss your options with your care team.

Chemotherapy

Chemotherapy (chemo) is a type of drug therapy used to treat cancer. It works by killing fast-growing cells in the body. Chemotherapy is used to destroy cancer cells, but it can also affect healthy, fast-growing cells like hair.

There are a variety of chemotherapy drugs. Some chemotherapy drugs kill abnormal cells, while others stop new cells from being made.

Chemotherapy drugs are liquids that are injected into a vein with a needle, or a pill that is swallowed. In most cases, chemotherapy is given in cycles of treatment days followed by days of rest. This allows the body to recover before the next cycle.

Cycles vary in length depending on which chemotherapy is used. You will have tests to see how well the treatment is working. You might spend time in the hospital during treatment.

Below are some examples of chemotherapies used to treat MDS:

- Azacitidine (Vidaza)
- Decitabine (Dacogen)
- Oral decitabine and cedazuridine (Inqovi)

These drugs are a type of chemotherapy called hypomethylating agents. They work by blocking DNA that helps abnormal cells grow. This helps to "turn on" genes that promote the growth of normal, healthy cells in the bone marrow.

Immunosuppressive therapy

Immunosuppressive therapy (IST) is a type of drug therapy that lowers the body's immune response to allow bone marrow stem cells to grow and make new blood cells.

Three IST drugs are used to treat MDS, usually hypocellular MDS with associated clinical features:

- Antithymocyte globulin (Atgam)
- Cyclosporin A
- Eltrombopag (Promacta)

Antithymocyte globulin

Antithymocyte globulin (ATG) is a drug used to treat MDS or reduce rejection after a bone marrow transplant. ATG works by decreasing your body's natural defense (immune system). This allows bone marrow to rebuild its supply of bone marrow stem cells, thus causing blood counts to go up.

Cyclosporin A

Cyclosporin A is a drug typically used in combination with ATG to treat acquired aplastic anemia, which is a condition where the immune system attacks the bone marrow. It is also used to prevent rejection after an organ transplant and to reduce immune response after a bone marrow transplant.

IDH inhibitors

Ivosidenib

Ivosidenib (Tibsovo) is a drug for people with MDS with *IDH1* mutations. The drug is a pill that, when taken, works by inhibiting the *IDH1* mutation. Some people with MDS who take this drug are able to be weaned off infusion therapy, which is a type of therapy that uses a needle placed into a vein, after 6 months of taking this pill.

Erythroid maturation agents

Eltrombopag

Eltrombopag (Promacta) is a drug used to treat adults with low blood platelet counts due to chronic immune thrombocytopenia (ITP) when other medicines have not worked. The drug increases the growth and development of platelets in the bone marrow. It is used for people with low platelet levels who also have either aplastic anemia, chronic immune thrombocytopenia, or chronic hepatitis C-associated thrombocytopenia.

Imetelstat

Imetelstat (Rytelo) is a drug for patients with lower-risk MDS who rely on transfusions to treat their anemia. Imetelstat works by targeting the genetic material of cancerous cells. By targeting this genetic material, the cells can’t create new cells or survive on their own, so they die.

Luspatercept-aamt

Luspatercept-aamt (Reblozyl) is a drug used to treat anemia in people with lower-risk MDS. It works by helping immature red blood cells develop and become mature, functional red blood cells. As a result, this increases hemoglobin levels in the bloodstream, which improves anemia in people with lower-risk MDS and anemia.

Immunomodulators

Lenalidomide

Lenalidomide (Revlimid) is a drug used to increase hemoglobin levels. Hemoglobin is the protein in red blood cells that carry oxygen. Lenalidomide is used to treat MDS with cells that are missing part of chromosome 5.

Chromosome 5 controls the amount of red blood cells that a person might have, which in turn controls how much hemoglobin a person has. When this chromosome is partially missing, it's referred to as "del(5q)." Lenalidomide might reduce the amount of transfusions that people with MDS with del(5q) need to get.

Hematopoietic cell transplant

Hematopoietic cell transplant (HCT), also called bone marrow transplant or stem cell transplant, is a type of treatment that uses chemotherapy to destroy cells in the bone marrow and then replaces them with new, healthy blood-forming cells ("hematopoietic" means "blood-forming.") The healthy blood stem cells will grow, form new bone marrow and blood cells, and attack remaining cancer cells.

For the treatment of MDS, blood stem cells from a donor are used for the transplant. This is called an allogeneic HCT (allo-HCT). Before the transplant, special testing must be done to make sure the donor is a good match for you. Human leukocyte antigen (HLA) typing is used to find a person's tissue type, called an HLA type.

Treatment steps for allogeneic HCT are described next.

Conditioning treatment

Before the transplant, you will receive high doses of strong (high-intensity) chemotherapy. Reduced-intensity regimens may also be available. This chemotherapy is referred to as conditioning treatment since it prepares, or conditions, your body to receive the donated blood stem cells.

Chemotherapy destroys normal cells and cancer cells in your bone marrow. It also greatly weakens your immune system so that your body doesn't kill the transplanted blood stem cells.

Radiation therapy may also be given as part of conditioning treatment.

Hematopoietic stem cell transfusion

After the conditioning treatment, the blood stem cells will be put into your body as a transfusion. A transfusion is a slow injection of blood products into a large vein. This process can take several hours to complete.

The transplanted blood stem cells will then travel to your bone marrow and grow. They will make new, healthy blood cells. This is called engraftment. It usually takes about 2 to 4 weeks.

Until then you will have little or no immune defense. This will put you at high risk for infection and bleeding. It may take a few weeks or months for blood cells to fully recover and for your immune system to return to normal.

Clinical trials

Clinical trials study how safe and helpful tests and treatments are for people. Clinical trials find out how to prevent, diagnose, and treat a disease like cancer. Because of clinical trials, providers find safe and helpful ways to improve your care and treatment of cancer.

Clinical trials have 4 phases.

- Phase I trials aim to find the safest and best dose of a new drug. Another aim is to find the best way to give the drug with the fewest side effects.
- Phase II trials assess if a drug works for a specific type of cancer.
- Phase III trials compare a new drug to a standard treatment.
- Phase IV trials track a drug's effectiveness over time after it has been approved for use.

To join a clinical trial, you must meet the conditions of the study. Patients in a clinical trial often are alike in terms of their cancer and general health. This helps to ensure that any change is from the treatment and not because of differences between patients.

If you decide to join a clinical trial, you will need to review and sign a paper called an informed consent form. This form describes the study in detail, including the risks and benefits. Even after you sign a consent form, you can stop taking part in a clinical trial at any time.

Ask your treatment team if there is an open clinical trial that you can join. There may be clinical trials where you get treatment or at nearby treatment centers. Discuss the risks and benefits of joining a clinical trial with your care team. Together, decide if a clinical trial is right for you.

Supportive care

Supportive care is the cornerstone of all MDS treatments. Supportive care aims to improve your quality of life by reducing symptoms from low blood counts. It includes care for health issues caused by cancer or cancer treatment.

It is sometimes referred to as "palliative care," but don't let that term scare you or limit your thinking. Supportive care is for everyone.

Supportive care options for MDS are described next and listed in **Guide 4.**

General health monitoring

All cancer treatments can cause unwanted health issues. Such health issues are called side effects. Side effects depend on many factors. These factors include the drug type and dose, length of treatment, and the person. Some side effects may be harmful to your health. Others may just be unpleasant.

Ask your treatment team for a complete list of side effects of your treatments. Also, tell your treatment team about any new or worsening symptoms. There may be ways to help you feel better and to prevent some side effects before they happen or get worse.

Psychosocial support

Distress is normal, common, and expected. Common symptoms include sadness, fear, and helplessness. Distress ranges from mild to extreme levels. Everyone with cancer has some level of distress at some point in time. Some people are more likely to be distressed than others.

Guide 4 Supportive care options
Monitoring for changes in general health
Psychosocial support
Quality-of-life assessment
Transfusions
Antibiotics for bacterial infections
Aminocaproic acid or other antifibrinolytic agents for bleeding
Iron chelation
Cytokines
Granulocyte colony-stimulated factor (G-CSF)

Those with uncontrolled symptoms, financial problems, lack of support, or a history of mental illness are likely to be distressed. People with psychosocial concerns are often helped by social work, counseling, or mental health services.

For more information, read the *NCCN Guidelines for Patients: Distress During Cancer Care*, available at NCCN.org/patientguidelines and on the Patient Guides for Cancer app.

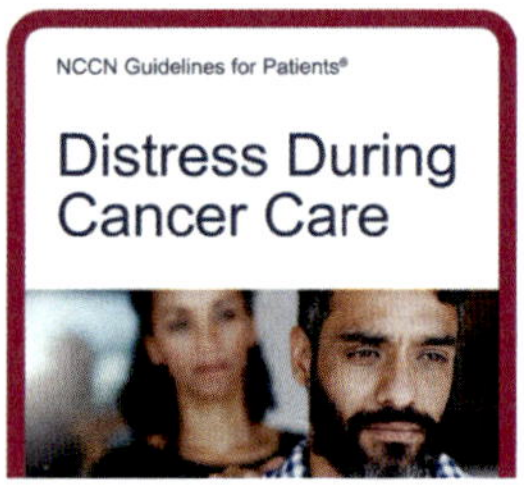

Quality-of-life assessment

A quality-of-life assessment is used to identify concerns early on such as pain or other problems that may be physical, psychosocial, and spiritual. There are several questionnaires available to your care team to evaluate quality of life, some even specific to MDS.

Transfusions

Low red blood cell counts caused by anemia may cause severe fatigue and other symptoms. People with MDS experiencing symptoms of anemia may benefit from a transfusion of red blood cells or platelets.

- Red blood cells – Transfusions of red blood cells may be needed to treat symptoms of anemia, such as shortness of breath or fatigue.
- Platelets – Transfusions of platelets may prevent or treat bleeding problems caused by having too few platelets. Transfusions are needed more frequently as platelets only survive for a few days.

Antibiotics for bacterial infections

Recurrent infections are one of the most common issues with MDS, after anemia. A low level of white blood cells increases your risk of infection. You should speak to your health care provider if there are any signs of infection, such as fever, pneumonia (cough, shortness of breath), or urinary tract infection (burning when urinating). You will likely be treated with antibiotics if you have bacterial infections.

Cytokines

Cytokines exist naturally in your body as part of your immune system. They can also be made in a laboratory to be used as cancer treatment. Cytokines trigger an immune response to attack cancer cells.

Cytokines used to treat MDS include epoetin alfa and granulocyte-colony stimulating factor (G-CSF). Epoetin alfa/darbepoetin alfa are used to treat a lower-than-normal number of red blood cells. G-CSF is a type of drug called a growth factor. It increases the number of blood cells in the blood. It can be used with chemotherapy, or before and after a stem cell transplant.

Aminocaproic acid

If your bleeding is not helped with a transfusion or a growth factor (such as darbepoetin alfa), then another option might be treatment with a drug called an antifibrinolytic agent, such as aminocaproic acid (Amicar).

Treatment team

Treating cancer takes a team approach. Some members of your care team will be with you throughout cancer treatment, others will only be there for certain parts of it. Get to know your care team and help them get to know you.

Depending on your diagnosis, your team might include the following specialists. Ask who will coordinate your care:

- **Your primary care provider** handles medical care not related to cancer. This person can help you express your feelings about treatments to your cancer care team.
- A **pathologist** interprets the cells, tissues, and organs removed during a biopsy or surgery.
- **A diagnostic radiologist** reads the results of x-rays and other imaging tests.
- **An interventional radiologist** performs needle biopsies, ablations, and arterially directed therapies, and places ports for treatment.
- **A surgical oncologist** performs operations to remove cancer.
- **A medical oncologist** treats cancer in adults using systemic therapy. Often, this person will lead the overall treatment team and keep track of tests and exams done by other specialists.
- **A radiation oncologist** prescribes and plans radiation therapy to treat cancer.
- **An anesthesiologist** gives anesthesia, a medicine so you do not feel pain during surgery or procedures.
- **A palliative care specialist** is an expert in the treatment of symptoms caused by cancer to improve a patient's quality of life and ease suffering.
- **Advanced practice providers** are registered nurse practitioners and physician assistants who monitor your health and provide care.
- **Oncology nurses** provide hands-on care, like giving systemic therapy, managing your care, answering questions, and helping you cope with side effects.
- **Nutritionists** can guide you on what foods or diets are most suitable for your particular condition.
- **Psychologists and psychiatrists** are mental health experts who can help manage issues such as depression, anxiety, or other mental health conditions that can affect how you feel.

Iron chelation

While transfusions help relieve symptoms of MDS or anemia, too many transfusions (20 or more), may cause iron to build up that can cause organ damage (iron overload). An overload of iron requires a special treatment to remove the excess iron.

This is called iron chelation. In iron chelation, drugs called chelating agents (deferoxamine as an injection under the skin or deferasirox as a pill) are used to bind with the iron so the body can get rid of it.

Key points

- Chemotherapy is used to destroy cancer cells, but it can also affect normal cells.
- Immunotherapy supports the body's natural defenses to fight myelodysplastic syndromes (MDS).
- The goal of a hematopoietic cell transplant (HCT) is to cure cancer by replacing unhealthy blood stem cells with healthy ones that will attack cancer cells.
- Supportive care is the cornerstone of all MDS treatments. Supportive care aims to improve your quality of life by reducing symptoms.
- Distress is normal, common, and expected.
- Get to know your care team and let them get to know you.

4
Treating lower-risk MDS

There is more than one treatment for lower-risk myelodysplastic syndrome (MDS). This chapter presents all of the treatment options recommended by NCCN MDS experts at this time.

Lower-risk myelodysplastic syndrome (MDS) is slow-growing and may not progress to acute myeloid leukemia (AML) for a long time. The goals in treating lower-risk MDS are to improve blood cell counts, reduce the need for blood transfusions, and improve quality of life.

Lower-risk MDS includes the following risk groups:

- IPSS-R very low, low, and intermediate
- WPSS very low, low, and intermediate
- IPSS-M very low, low, and moderate low

If you have one of these risk groups of MDS without symptoms, you may not need treatment right away. Instead, you will have regular check-ups and your blood counts will be checked. This is referred to as active monitoring or "watching and waiting."

However, if you have low-risk MDS with anemia and are having some symptoms, you may need treatment. Let's look at some of these treatment options below.

For more information about how any of these treatments work in your body, see *Chapter 3: Treating MDS*.

Low-risk MDS with anemia

Symptomatic anemia with del(5q) and low blasts

If you are experiencing symptoms of anemia and are found to have MDS with del(5q), treatment will be based on the level of erythropoietin (EPO) in the blood. EPO is a hormone produced mainly by the kidneys. It plays a key role in the production of red blood cells.

Serum EPO 500 mU/mL or less

MDS with low blasts, del(5q), and a serum EPO of 500 mU/mL or less is treated with lenalidomide (preferred treatment) or an erythropoiesis-stimulating agent, such as epoetin alfa (Procrit) or darbepoetin alfa (Aranesp).

Lenalidomide is a chemotherapy drug used to increase hemoglobin levels. Epoetin alfa/darbepoetin alfa is a synthetic form of erythropoietin used to treat anemia by increasing red blood cell production.

If neither of the treatments described above work for you, NCCN MDS experts recommend finding a clinical trial or your care team will prescribe you a chemotherapy such as azacitidine (Vidaza). Other options include chemotherapies like decitabine (Dacogen, as an infusion) or decitabine and cedazuridine (Inqovi, as an oral treatment), or an immunotherapy, imetelstat (Rytelo), depending on your health and age.

Low doses of azacitidine or decitabine have been shown to show some improvement for people with low-risk MDS. Oral decitabine and cedazuridine (Inqovi) can be used as a replacement for intravenous decitabine in patients at lower risk for MDS.

If you have an *IDH1* mutation and none of these treatments are working, then you may be prescribed the IDH1 inhibitor ivosidenib (Tibsovo). If you do not have an *IDH1* mutation, consider entering a clinical trial. Or depending on your health, you might be a candidate for a bone marrow transplant.

Serum EPO more than 500 mU/mL

MDS with low blasts, del(5q), and a serum EPO of 500 mU/mL or more is treated with lenalidomide, which is an immunomodulator.

If the treatment described above doesn't work for you, NCCN MDS experts recommend finding a clinical trial or your care team will prescribe you azacitidine (Vidaza), which is a chemotherapy.

Other options include chemotherapies like decitabine (Dacogen, as an infusion) or decitabine and cedazuridine (Inqovi, as an oral treatment), or an immunotherapy, imetelstat (Rytelo), depending on your health and age.

Low doses of azacitidine or decitabine have been shown to show some improvement for people with low-risk MDS. Oral decitabine and cedazuridine (Inqovi) can be used as a replacement for intravenous decitabine in patients at lower risk for MDS.

If you have an *IDH1* mutation and none of these treatments are working, then you may be prescribed the IDH1 inhibitor ivosidenib (Tibsovo). If you do not have an *IDH1* mutation, consider entering a clinical trial. Or depending on your health, you might be a candidate for a bone marrow transplant.

Symptomatic anemia with low blasts and *SF3B1* mutation

If you have a *SF3B1* mutation and there are low blasts, you may receive luspatercept-aamt (Reblozyl), which is an erythroid maturation agent. Or you may receive imetelstat (Rytelo), which is an immunotherapy. If there is no response on the imetelstat, you'll be started on lenalidomide, which is an immunomodulator.

If there's no response on luspatercept-aamt, the next treatment depends on the serum EPO. See below for more information. For more information on treatment for MDS with *SF3B1*, **see Guide 5** on the next page.

Serum EPO 500 mU/mL or less

MDS with *SF3B1* and serum EPO of 500 mU/mL or less is treated with imetelstat (Rytelo), which is an immunotherapy.

Other recommended treatments include an erythropoiesis-stimulating agent, such as epoetin alfa or darbepoetin alfa, with or without a granulocyte colony-stimulating factor (G-CSF). Epoetin alfa/darbepoetin alfa is a synthetic form of EPO used to treat anemia by increasing red blood cell production. G-CSF drives the bone marrow to make additional neutrophils or granulocytes and decrease the risk for infection. This drug can be used with chemotherapy, or before or after stem cell transplant.

If neither of the treatments described above work for you, NCCN MDS experts recommend finding a clinical trial or your care team will prescribe you azacitidine (Vidaza), which is a chemotherapy. Other options include chemotherapies like decitabine (Dacogen, as

Guide 5
Symptomatic anemia with no del(5q) and an *SF3B1* mutation

Serum EPO 500 mU/mL or less	Preferred: Epoetin alfa Darbepoetin alfa Other recommended: Luspatercept-aamt	→ **If no response or loss of response, the options are:** • Imetelstat (preferred) • Epoetin alfa with or without G-CSF or lenalidomide • Darbepoetin alfa with or without G-CSF or lenalidomide • Luspatercept-aamt (if not previously used)	→ **If no response after 4 months**: Imetelstat (if not previously used) Follow serum EPO 500 mU/mL or more If *IDH1* mutation, ivosidenib
Serum EPO more than 500 mU/mL	Good probability to respond to IST	→ Treat with ATG with or without cyclosporin A or eltrombopag	→ If no response or intolerance, see row below
	Poor probability to respond to IST	→ **Treatment options:** • Clinical trial • Azacitidine • Decitabine • Imetelstat • Decitabine-cedazuridine • Consider lenalidomide	→ **If no response with 6 cycles of azacitidine or 4 cycles of decitabine or intolerance,** if no *IDH1* mutation: • Clinical trial • Consider allo-HCT in some cases If *IDH1* mutation, ivosidenib

an infusion), or decitabine and cedazuridine (Inqovi, as an oral treatment).

Low doses of azacitidine or decitabine have been shown to show some improvement for people with low-risk MDS. Oral decitabine and cedazuridine (Inqovi) can be used as a replacement for intravenous decitabine in patients at lower risk for MDS.

If you have an *IDH1* mutation and none of these treatments are working, then you may be prescribed the IDH1 inhibitor ivosidenib (Tibsovo). If you do not have an *IDH1* mutation, consider entering a clinical trial. Or depending on your health, you might be a candidate for a bone marrow transplant.

Serum EPO more than 500 mU/mL
MDS with low blasts and serum EPO more than 500 mU/mL may be treated with lenalidomide, which is an immunomodulator.

If this treatment doesn't work for you, NCCN MDS experts recommend finding a clinical trial or your care team will prescribe you azacitidine (Vidaza), which is a chemotherapy. Other options include chemotherapies like decitabine (Dacogen, as an infusion) and decitabine and cedazuridine (Inqovi, as an oral treatment), or an immunotherapy, imetelstat (Rytelo), depending on your health and age.

Low doses of azacitidine or decitabine have been shown to show some improvement for people with low-risk MDS. Oral decitabine and cedazuridine (Inqovi) can be used as a replacement for intravenous decitabine in patients at lower risk for MDS.

If you have an *IDH1* mutation and none of these treatments are working, then you may be prescribed the IDH1 inhibitor ivosidenib (Tibsovo). If you do not have an *IDH1* mutation, consider entering a clinical trial. Or depending on your health, you might be a candidate for a bone marrow transplant.

Symptomatic anemia with no del(5q) and other cytogenetic abnormalities

Serum EPO 500 mU/mL or less
MDS with no del(5q) and serum EPO of 500 mU/mL or less is treated with an erythropoiesis-stimulating agent, such as epoetin alfa or darbepoetin alfa. Another recommended treatment is luspatercept-aamt.

If there's no response, the care team may switch the medications to another recommended agent or to imetelstat (Rytelo), which is an immunotherapy. Your team may add a G-CSF or lenalidomide (Revlimid) to the regimen.

G-CSF drives the bone marrow to make additional neutrophils or granulocytes and decreases the risk of infection. This drug can be used with chemotherapy, or before or after a stem cell transplant.

If none of those treatments described above work for you, NCCN MDS experts recommend finding a clinical trial. Or your care team may prescribe you azacitidine (Vidaza), which is a chemotherapy. Other options include chemotherapies like decitabine (Dacogen, as an infusion) and decitabine and cedazuridine (Inqovi, as an oral treatment), or an immunotherapy, imetelstat (Rytelo), depending on your health and age.

Low doses of azacitidine or decitabine can show some improvement for people with low-risk MDS. Oral decitabine and cedazuridine (Inqovi) can be used as a replacement for intravenous decitabine in patients at lower risk for MDS.

If you have an *IDH1* mutation and none of these treatments are working, then you may be prescribed the IDH1 inhibitor ivosidenib (Tibsovo). If you do not have an *IDH1* mutation, consider entering a clinical trial. Or depending on your health, you might be a candidate for a bone marrow transplant.

Serum EPO more than 500 mU/mL

MDS with serum EPO more than 500 mU/mL is treated based on the probability of responding to immunosuppressive therapy (IST). IST is used to treat people 60 years of age or under who have 5 percent (5%) or less marrow blasts.

If there is a good chance for a response to the IST, treatment will also include antithymocyte globulin (ATG) with or without cyclosporin A and/or eltrombopag (Promacta).

ATG is a drug used to treat MDS or reduce rejection after a bone marrow transplant.

ATG works by decreasing your body's natural defense (immune system). This allows bone marrow to rebuild its supply of bone marrow stem cells, causing blood counts to go up.

Cyclosporin A is used to prevent organ rejection after transplant. Eltrombopag is used to treat low platelet counts in the bloodstream.

If there is a poor chance of responding to IST, treatment options include:

- Clinical trial
- Azacitidine (Vidaza)
- Decitabine (Dacogen)
- Imetelstat (Rytelo)
- Oral decitabine-cedazuridine (Inqovi)
- Lenalidomide (Revlimid), if needed

If you have an *IDH1* mutation and none of these treatments are working, then you may be prescribed the IDH1 inhibitor ivosidenib (Tibsovo). If you do not have an *IDH1* mutation, consider entering a clinical trial. Or depending on your health, you might be a candidate for a bone marrow transplant.

Low-risk MDS without anemia

If you have thrombocytopenia, neutropenia, or increased marrow blasts you will be treated by hypomethylating agents such as azacitidine (Vidaza), decitabine (Dacogen), decitabine-cedazuridine (Inqovi), IST in certain cases (with or without eltrombopag), or clinical trial. IST is used to treat people aged 60 years or under who have 5 percent (5%) or less marrow blasts.

If there is no response or your disease worsens, your health care provider will consider other recommended medicines, a clinical trial, or a bone marrow transplant. If you have an *IDH1* mutation, you might receive ivosidenib.

For more information, **see Guide 6.**

Key points

- The goals in treating low-risk MDS are to improve blood cell counts, lessen the need for blood transfusions, and improve quality of life.
- Treatment options are based on factors such as the MDS subtype, risk score, as well as your age and health status.
- Talk to your provider about treatment options based on your type of MDS and the possible risks and benefits.
- If you have symptomatic anemia, treatment options will be based on the presence of del(5q) and blast count.
- A clinical trial is a good option for treating low-risk MDS when other options aren't possible.

Guide 6
Thrombocytopenia, neutropenia, or increased marrow blasts

Treatment options include:	• Clinical trial • Azacitidine (preferred) • Decitabine • Oral decitabine-cedazuridine • IST (with or without eltrombopag)
If disease progression or no response, then:	• Consider hypomethylating agents • Clinical trial • Consider HCT
If *IDH1* mutation, then:	• Ivosidenib

5
Treating higher-risk MDS

People with higher-risk MDS are more likely to have problems from the disease and progress to acute myeloid leukemia (AML) in a shorter period of time. The goals of treatment for higher-risk myelodysplastic syndromes (MDS) are to slow or stop MDS from turning into AML and to help people live longer.

In high-risk myelodyplastic syndromes (MDS), immature cells called blast cells often make up more than 5 percent (5%) of the cells in the bone marrow. People with high-risk disease are more likely to have multiple types of low blood counts (cytopenias), anemia (low hemoglobin), neutropenia (low white blood cell counts), and/or thrombocytopenia (low platelets).

In high-risk MDS, people are more likely to require blood or platelet transfusions and treatment for infections.

High-risk MDS includes the following risk groups:

- IPSS-R intermediate, high, and very high
- WPSS high and very high
- IPSS-M moderate-high, high, and very high

Treatment

Treatment options for high-risk MDS depend on treatment goals. Treatment goals include potential cure or disease control. If the goal is cure, then an allogeneic hematopoietic cell transplant (allo-HCT), also known as a bone marrow transplant, will be recommended.

Depending on a person's age and the stage or status of MDS, there may or may not be additional treatment before qualifying for allo-HCT. Treatment options are shown further in **Guide 7.**

Not everyone is a candidate for a stem cell transplant. Treatment options differ based on your age, your health, and your treatment goals.

Transplant candidate

If you are a transplant candidate, treatment options will include:

- Allo-HCT
- Azacitidine followed by allo-HCT
- Decitabine followed by allo-HCT
- Oral decitabine-cedazuridine followed by allo-HCT
- High-intensity chemotherapy followed by allo-HCT
- Clinical trial, followed by allo-HCT

Allogeneic hematopoietic cell transplant

An allogeneic hematopoietic cell transplant (allo-HCT) is used in treating MDS. In this procedure, a person receives blood-forming stem cells from a donor.

For best results, the donor's cell type (also known as the human leukocyte antigen [HLA] type) is matched to the person receiving the transplant. Donors may include a sibling, parent, or child. Less often, the donor is not related.

When treatment is needed in addition to allo-HCT, azacitidine (Vidaza) decitabine (Dacogen), decitabine-cedazuridine (Inqovi), or high-intensity chemotherapy is used.

Azacitidine and decitabine are hypomethylating agents. Hypomethylating agents are a type of chemotherapy that block methyl groups from binding to DNA. They turn silenced genes back on, which allows blasts to mature and develop into healthy cells.

High-intensity therapy includes intensive induction chemotherapy or allo-HCT. High-intensity chemotherapy refers to the delivery of chemotherapy before definitive surgery or radiation therapy.

If you have a mutation in the *IDH1* gene, then you may receive ivosidenib before allo-HCT.

Treatment relapse

If there's no response to the medicine or a relapse following a successful treatment, the next course of therapy is to consider a clinical

Guide 7
Treatment options based on transplant status

If transplant candidate	**Treatment options include:** Allo-HCT Azacitidine followed by allo-HCT Decitabine followed by allo-HCT Oral decitabine-cedazuridine followed by allo-HCT High-intensity chemotherapy followed by allo-HCT Clinical trial followed by allo-HCT	**If relapse after allo-HCT or no response, then:** Consider allo-HCT or donor lymphocyte infusion Azacitidine Decitabine Clinical trial Supportive care
If not transplant candidate	**Treatment options include:** Azacitidine (preferred) Decitabine Decitabine-cedazuridine Clinical trial Clinical trial followed by allo-HCT	**If no response or relapse, then:** Clinical trial If *IDH1* mutation, ivosidenib Clinical trial

trial or try one of the hypomethylating agents (azacitidine, decitabine, or oral decitabine-cedazuridine) that haven't been tried before.

Not a transplant candidate

If you are not a candidate for a stem cell transplant, treatment options include:

- Clinical trial
- Azacitidine (Vidaza)
- Decitabine (Dacogen)
- Oral decitabine and cedazuridine (Inqovi)

If there is a response to treatment, the treatment will continue. If there is no response or a relapse, options include a clinical trial or supportive care. A relapse occurs when MDS comes back after treatment. This can happen at any point (weeks, months, or even years) after the first cancer was treated.

If you have an *IDH1* mutation in addition and none of these treatments are working, then you may be prescribed the IDH1 inhibitor ivosidenib (Tibsovo). If you do not have an *IDH1* mutation, consider entering a clinical trial. Or depending on your health, you might be a candidate for a bone marrow transplant.

Key points

- High-risk myelodysplastic syndrome (MDS) is more likely to grow faster and progress to acute myeloid leukemia (AML) in a shorter period of time.
- In high-risk MDS, immature cells called blast cells often make up more than 5 percent (5%) of the cells in the bone marrow.
- Treatment options for high-risk MDS depend on treatment goals. Treatment goals include potential cure or disease control.
- An allogeneic hematopoietic cell transplant (allo-HCT) is typically used in treating MDS.

6
MDS/MPN overlap syndromes

Some people may show signs of both myelodysplastic syndromes (MDS) and myeloproliferative neoplasms (MPN). These are referred to as MDS/MPN overlap syndromes. This chapter explains the different overlap syndromes and how they're treated.

Myelodysplastic syndromes (MDS) are a group of diseases where the bone marrow does not make enough healthy mature blood cells (red blood cells, white blood cells, and platelets).

Myeloproliferative neoplasms (MPN) are a group of diseases where the body makes too many of one or more types of blood cells.

MDS can overlap with MPN. These are called myeloid disorders.

Myeloid disorders have dysplastic (abnormal cells) and proliferative (increased numbers of cells) features. These disorders are not considered to be MDS or MPN, because they have some features of both syndromes.

NCCN considers myeloid disorders to be a subtype of MDS in its clinical guidelines, but if you need to know more about MPN specifically, read the *NCCN Guidelines for Patients: Myeloproliferative Neoplasms*, available at NCCN.org/patientguidelines and on the Patient Guides for Cancer app.

Subtypes of MDS/MPN

The following are subtypes of MDS/MPN:

- Chronic myelomonocytic leukemia (CMML)
- MDS/MPN and neutrophilia
- MDS/MPN, not otherwise specified (NOS)
- MDS/MPN with *SF3B1* mutation and thrombocytosis

CMML

Chronic myelomonocytic leukemia (CMML) is a disease in which too many monocytes, a type of white blood cell, develop in the bone marrow. Some of the cells do not develop into mature white blood cells.

The monocytes and immature blood cells (called blasts) overwhelm the other cells in the bone marrow so there are not enough red blood cells and platelets.

The World Health Organization (WHO) categorizes CMML into 2 subtypes based on the number of blasts in the blood and bone marrow:

- CMML-1 means that 10 percent (10%) or less of the cells in the bone marrow are blasts.
- CMML-2 means that 20 percent (20%) or less of the cells in the bone marrow are blasts.

MDS/MPN and neutrophilia

MDS/MPN and neutrophilia is a rare disorder where too many blood stem cells in the bone marrow develop into granulocytes (a type of white blood cell). Neutrophilia is defined as having too many granulocytes in the blood.

Some of the granulocytes do not mature. Immature blood cells are called blasts. Gradually the blasts and granulocytes overwhelm healthy red blood cells and platelets in the bone marrow.

MDS/MPN, not otherwise specified

MDS/MPN, not otherwise specified (NOS), is a rare disorder where too many stem cells in the bone marrow develop into blood cells (red blood cells, white blood cells, or platelets). Some of the blood cells do not mature. Immature blood cells are called blasts. Gradually the blasts and abnormal cells crowd out the healthy blood cells in the bone marrow.

MDS/MPN with *SF3B1* mutation and thrombocytosis

MDS/MPN with *SF3B1* mutation and thrombocytosis is a disorder with a high level of one or more types of blood cells in the blood and bone marrow. In this subtype, at least 15 percent (15%) of immature blood cells in the bone marrow are ring sideroblasts with a high platelet count (greater than or equal to 450,000).

Treatment

Treatment options are based on the subtype of MDS/MPN disorder. Options range from observation to hypomethylating agents (HMAs), such as azacitidine and decitabine, to allogeneic hematopoietic cell transplant (allogenic HCT, also referred to as bone marrow transplant or stem cell transplant).

For information on specific subtypes and their treatment options, **see Guide 8.**

Key points

- Myelodysplastic syndromes (MDS) is a group of diseases in which bone marrow does not make enough healthy mature blood cells (red blood cells, white blood cells, and platelets).
- In myeloproliferative neoplasms (MPN), the body makes too many of one or more types of blood cells.
- MDS can overlap with MPN. These are called myeloid disorders.
- Treatment options are based on the MDS/MPN subtype. Speak with your health care provider to determine the best treatment option for you.

Guide 8
MDS/MPN overlap management

Subtype	Common mutations	Treatment
CMML-1	*TET2, SRSF2, ASXL1, RUNX1, NRAS, CBL*	Consider HMA or hydroxyurea
CMML-2	*TET2, SRSF2, ASXL1, RUNX1, NRAS, CBL*	HMA with or without venetoclax and/or allogeneic HCT
MDS/MPN and neutrophilia	*SETBP1, ETNK1, BCR::ABL1* negative	Consider HMA and/or ruxolitinib and/or allogeneic HCT
MDS/MPN, not otherwise specified (NOS)	*TET2, NRAS, RUNX1, CBL, SETBP1, ASXL1*	Consider HMA and/or allogeneic HCT
MDS/MPN with *SF3B1* mutation and thrombocytosis	*SF3B1, JAK2, MPL, CALR*	Consider HMA and/or lenalidomide or luspatercept-aamt

7
Making treatment decisions

It's important to be comfortable with the cancer treatment you choose. This choice starts with having an open and honest conversation with your care team.

It's your choice

In shared decision-making, you and your care team share information, discuss the options, and agree on a treatment plan. It starts with an open and honest conversation between you and your care team.

Treatment decisions are very personal. What is important to you may not be important to someone else. Some things that may play a role in your decision-making:

- What you want and how that might differ from what others want
- Your religious and spiritual beliefs
- Your feelings about certain treatments
- Your feelings about pain or side effects
- Cost of treatment, travel to treatment centers, and time away from school or work
- Quality of life and length of life
- How active you are and the activities that are important to you

Think about what you want from treatment. Discuss openly the risks and benefits of specific treatments and procedures. Weigh options and share concerns with your care team. If you take the time to build a relationship with your care team, it will help you feel supported when considering options and making treatment decisions.

Second opinion

It is normal to want to start treatment as soon as possible. While cancer can't be ignored, there is time to have another doctor review your test results and suggest a treatment plan. This is called getting a second opinion, and it's a normal part of cancer care. Even doctors get second opinions!

Things you can do to prepare:

- Check with your insurance company about its rules on second opinions. There may be out-of-pocket costs to see doctors who are not part of your insurance plan.
- Make plans to have copies of all your records sent to the doctor you will see for your second opinion.

Support groups

Many people diagnosed with cancer find support groups to be helpful. Support groups often include people at different stages of treatment. Some people may be newly diagnosed, while others may be finished with treatment. If your hospital or community doesn't have support groups for people with cancer, check out the websites listed in this book.

Questions to ask

Possible questions to ask your care team are listed on the following pages. Feel free to use these questions or come up with your own.

Questions about cancer testing

1. What tests will I have?
2. Do the tests have any risks?
3. Will my insurance pay for all of the tests you are recommending?
4. Do I need to do anything to prepare for testing?
5. Should I bring someone with me to the appointments?
6. Where do I go for testing, and how long will it take?
7. If any of the tests will hurt, what will you do to make me comfortable?
8. How soon will I know the results and who will explain them to me?
9. How can I get a copy of the pathology report and other test results?
10. Is there an online portal with my test results?

Questions about treatment options

1. What are my treatment options?
2. Is a clinical trial an option for me?
3. What will happen if I do nothing?
4. Are you suggesting options other than what NCCN recommends? If yes, why?
5. How do my age, sex, overall health, and other factors affect my options?
6. What if I am pregnant, or planning to become pregnant?
7. Does any option offer a cure or long-term cancer control?
8. What are the side effects of the treatments?
9. How do I get a second opinion?
10. How long do I have to decide about treatment, and is there a social worker or someone who can help me decide?

Questions about resources and support

1. Who can I talk to about help with housing, food, and other basic needs?
2. What assistance is available for transportation, childcare, and home care?
3. Who can tell me what my options for health insurance are and assist me with applying for insurance coverage?
4. How much will I have to pay for my treatment? What help is available to pay for medicines and other treatment?
5. Who can help me with my concerns about work or school?
6. How can I connect with others and build a support system?
7. Who can I talk to if I don't feel safe at home, at work, or in my neighborhood?

Questions about what to expect

1. Does this hospital or cancer center offer the best treatment for me?
2. Do I have a choice of when to begin treatment?
3. How long will treatment last?
4. Will my insurance cover the treatment you're recommending?
5. Are there any programs to help pay for treatment?
6. What supportive care and services are available to me and my caregivers?
7. Who should I contact with questions or concerns if the office is closed?
8. How will you know if treatment is working?
9. What are the chances of the cancer worsening or returning?
10. What follow-up care is needed after treatment?

Questions about side effects

1. What are the possible complications and side effects of treatment?
2. Does the cancer itself cause any side effects?
3. Which side effects are most common and how long do they usually last?
4. Which side effects are serious or life-threatening?
5. Are there any long-term or permanent side effects?
6. What symptoms should I report right away, and who do I contact?
7. What can I do to prevent or relieve the side effects of treatment?
8. Do any medications worsen side effects?
9. Do any side effects lessen or worsen in severity over time?
10. Will you stop or change treatment if there are serious side effects?

Questions about clinical trials

1. Do you recommend that I consider a clinical trial for treatment?
2. How do I find clinical trials that I can participate in?
3. What are the treatments used in the clinical trial?
4. Has the treatment been used for other types of cancer?
5. What are the risks and benefits of this treatment?
6. What side effects should I expect and how will they be managed?
7. How long will I be in the clinical trial?
8. Will I be able to get other treatment if this doesn't work?
9. How will you know if the treatment is working?
10. Will the clinical trial cost me anything?

Questions about your care team's experience

1. Are you board certified? If yes, in what area?
2. What is your experience as well as your team's experience with treating the type of cancer I have?
3. How many patients like me (of the same age, gender, race) have you treated?
4. Will you be consulting with experts to discuss my care? Whom will you consult?
5. Is this treatment (or procedure) a major part of your practice? How often have you done this treatment (or procedure) in the last year?
6. How many of your patients have had complications? What were the complications?

Resources

BMT InfoNet
bmtinfonet.org

CancerCare
Cancercare.org

Imerman Angels
Imermanangels.org

Leukemia Research Foundation
Leukemiarf.org

MDS Foundation
MDS-Foundation.org

National Bone Marrow Transplant Link (nbmtLINK)
nbmtlink.org

National Coalition for Cancer Survivorship
canceradvocacy.org

NMDP
nmdp.org/one-on-one

The Leukemia & Lymphoma Society
LLS.org/PatientSupport

Triage Cancer
Triagecancer.org

We want your feedback!

Our goal is to provide helpful and easy-to-understand information on cancer.

Take our survey to let us know what we got right and what we could do better.

NCCN.org/patients/feedback

Words to know

acute myeloid leukemia (AML)
A fast-growing cancer that starts in the bone marrow and causes too many immature white blood cells to be made.

allogeneic hematopoietic cell transplant (allo-HCT)
A treatment in which the patient receives healthy, immature blood-forming cells from another person to replace damaged or diseased cells in the bone marrow.

anemia
A condition in which the number of red blood cells is low.

biopsy
Removal of small amounts of tissue from the body to be tested for disease.

blast cell
An immature blood cell.

blood cell growth factors
Substances that increase the production of new blood cells in the bone marrow.

blood smear
A test in which a drop of blood is placed on a slide and viewed with a microscope to assess the size, shape, type, and maturity of the blood cells.

blood stem cell
An immature blood-forming cell from which all other types of blood cells are made. Also called hematopoietic stem cell.

bone marrow
The soft, sponge-like tissue in the center of most bones where blood cells are made.

bone marrow aspiration
The removal of a small amount of liquid bone marrow to test for disease.

bone marrow biopsy
The removal of a small amount of solid bone and bone marrow to test for disease.

chemotherapy
Treatment with drugs that kill abnormal cells or stop new ones from being made.

chromosomes
Long strands that contain bundles of coded instructions for making and controlling cells.

clinical trial
Research on a test or treatment to assess its safety or how well it works.

complete blood count (CBC)
A test of the number of blood cells in a sample.

conditioning treatment
Treatment that is used to destroy cells in the bone marrow to prepare (condition) the body for a hematopoietic cell transplant.

cytogenetic testing
A test that uses a microscope to examine a cell's chromosomes.

cytopenia
A condition in which the number of blood cells is low.

del(5q)
An abnormal chromosome change in which the "q" part of chromosome 5 is missing (deleted).

DNA
A chain of chemicals that contains coded instructions for making and controlling cells.

differential
Measurement of the different types of white blood cells present in a blood sample.

donor
A person who gives their organs, tissues, or cells to another person.

dysplasia
The presence of cells with an abnormal size, shape, or look (appearance) when viewed with a microscope.

erythropoietin (EPO)
A natural substance in the body that tells (stimulates) the bone marrow to make more red blood cells.

fatigue
Severe tiredness despite getting enough sleep that limits one's ability to function.

flow cytometry
A test that looks at certain substances on the surface of cells to identify the type of cells present.

fluorescence in situ hybridization (FISH)
A lab test that uses special dyes to look for abnormal changes in a cell's genes and chromosomes.

folate
A nutrient in the body that is needed to make red blood cells.

gene
A set of coded instructions in cells for making and controlling cells.

gene mutation
An abnormal change in the coded instructions in cells for making and controlling cells.

genetic tests
Tests of the coded instructions in cells that are needed to make and control cells.

granulocyte colony-stimulating factor (G-CSF)
A substance that helps (stimulates) the bone marrow to make more white blood cells called neutrophils. It is made naturally in the body but can also be made in a lab.

hematopoietic cell transplant (HCT)
A treatment that replaces damaged or diseased cells in the bone marrow with healthy blood-forming cells. Also called stem cell transplant.

hematopoietic stem cell or hematopoietic cell
An immature blood-forming cell from which all other types of blood cells are made. Also called blood stem cell.

hemoglobin
A protein in red blood cells that carries oxygen.

high-intensity chemotherapy
Treatment with high doses of strong cancer drugs; typically used to destroy cells in the bone marrow to prepare (condition) the body for a hematopoietic cell transplant..

high-intensity treatment
Treatment that is more likely to cause severe side effects and often requires a hospital stay.

high-risk MDS
MDS that is more likely to progress faster or turn quickly into acute myeloid leukemia (AML) if not treated.

hormone
A chemical in the body that activates cells or organs.

human leukocyte antigen (HLA)
Special proteins on the surface of cells that help the body to tell its own cells apart from foreign cells.

human leukocyte antigen (HLA) typing
A blood test that finds a person's HLA type—the unique set of proteins on the surface of cells that help the body to tell its own cells apart from foreign cells.

immune response
The action of the body's natural defense against infections and disease in response to foreign substances.

immune system
The body's natural defense against infection and disease.

immunomodulators
Drugs that change (modify) different parts of the immune system.

immunosuppressive therapy (IST)
Treatment with drugs that weaken (suppress) the body's immune system.

immunotherapy
Treatment with drugs that modify the immune system to help the body fight cancer.

International Prognostic Scoring System Molecular (IPSS-M)
A system that health care providers use to rate the severity of MDS and classify it into groups based on the likely outcome (prognosis) and molecular features.

iron
A mineral that is found in red blood cells and that the body needs to make new red blood cells.

iron chelation therapy
Treatment that is used to remove excess iron from the body.

low-intensity chemotherapy
Treatment with cancer drugs that are less likely to cause severe side effects.

low-intensity treatment
Treatment that is less likely to cause severe side effects and usually does not require a hospital stay.

lower-risk myelodysplastic syndromes (MDS)
MDS that is more likely to grow slowly and may not cause many or severe symptoms for a long time.

lymphocyte
A type of white blood cell that helps protect the body from infection and disease.

molecular test
Tests that look for abnormal changes in genes known to have an effect on cancer treatment or outcomes.

monocyte
A type of white blood cell.

mutation
An abnormal change.

myeloproliferative neoplasm (MPN)
A cancer in which the bone marrow makes too many red blood cells, white blood cells, or platelets.

neutropenia
A condition in which the number of white blood cells called neutrophils is too low.

neutrophil
A type of white blood cell that helps fight infections and has small particles (granules).

platelet
A type of blood cell that helps control bleeding.

platelet transfusion
A slow injection of platelets—blood cells that help control bleeding—into a vein.

prognosis
The likely or expected course, pattern, and outcome of a disease.

prognostic factor
Something that affects and helps predict the likely pattern and outcome of a disease.

prognostic scoring system
A system that health care providers use to rate the severity of MDS and classify it into groups based on the likely outcome (prognosis).

recurrent gene mutation
Mutations that occur repeatedly, generally at some frequency.

red blood cell
A type of blood cell that carries oxygen from the lungs to the rest of the body.

red blood cell growth factor
A substance that increases the production of new red blood cells. It is made naturally in the body but can also be made in a lab to use as treatment.

red blood cell transfusion
A slow injection of red blood cells into a vein.

regimen
A treatment plan that specifies the dose, schedule, and duration of treatment.

relapse
The return or worsening of cancer after a period of improvement.

reticulocyte
Younger (precursor) cells that become mature red blood cells.

Revised International Prognostic Scoring System (IPSS-R)
A newer system that health care providers use to rate the severity of MDS and classify it into groups based on the likely outcome (prognosis).

ring sideroblasts
Young red blood cells that have too much iron and show up as a circle (ring) around the center of the cells.

risk group
Classification of MDS based on its severity and the chance (risk) that it will progress to AML (acute myeloid leukemia).

risk score
A rating of the severity of MDS that describes how fast or slow it will likely grow and progress.

serum EPO
The amount of natural erythropoietin—a substance made in the body that causes red blood cells to grow—that is found in the blood.

side effect
An unhealthy or unpleasant physical or emotional condition caused by treatment.

subtype
Smaller groups that a type of cancer is divided into based on certain features of the cancer cells.

supportive care
Treatment for the symptoms or health conditions caused by cancer or cancer treatment.

thrombocytopenia
A condition in which there is a low number of platelets—blood cells that help control bleeding.

transfusion
A slow injection of whole blood or parts of blood into a vein.

treatment response
An outcome or improvement in disease that is caused by treatment.

white blood cell
A type of blood cell that helps fight infections in the body.

white blood cell growth factor
A substance that increases the production of new white blood cells. It is made naturally in the body but can also be made in a lab to use as treatment.

WHO classification-based Prognostic Scoring System (WPSS)
A system that health care providers use to rate the severity of MDS and classify it into groups based on the likely outcome (prognosis).

NCCN Contributors

This patient guide is based on the NCCN Clinical Practice Guidelines in Oncology (NCCN Guidelines®) for Myelodysplastic Syndromes, Version 3.2024. It was adapted, reviewed, and published with help from the following people:

Dorothy A. Shead, MS
Senior Director
Patient Information Operations

Tim Rinehart, MS
Medical Writer

Laura Phillips
Graphic Artist

The NCCN Clinical Practice Guidelines in Oncology (NCCN Guidelines®) for Myelodysplastic Syndromes, Version 3.2024 were developed by the following NCCN Panel Members:

*Peter L. Greenberg, MD/Chair
Stanford Cancer Institute

Richard M. Stone, MD/Vice Chair
Dana-Farber/Brigham and Women's Cancer Center

Yasmin Abaza, MD
Robert H. Lurie Comprehensive Cancer Center of Northwestern University

Aref Al-Kali, MD
Mayo Clinic Comprehensive Cancer Center

Sarah Anand, MD
University of Michigan Rogel Cancer Center

John M. Bennett, MD
University of Rochester

Uma Borate, MD, MSc
The Ohio State University Comprehensive Cancer Center - James Cancer Hospital and Solove Research Institute

Andrew M. Brunner, MD
Mass General Cancer Center

Wanxing Chai-Ho, MD
UCLA Jonsson Comprehensive Cancer Center

Peter Curtin, MD
City of Hope National Medical Center

Carlos M. de Castro, MD
Duke Cancer Institute

H. Joachim Deeg, MD
Fred Hutchinson Cancer Research Center/ Seattle Cancer Care Alliance

Amy E. DeZern, MD, MHS
Johns Hopkins Kimmel Cancer Center

Shira Dinner, MD
Robert H. Lurie Comprehensive Cancer Center of Northwestern University

Karin Gaensler, MD
UCSF Helen Diller Family Comprehensive Cancer Center

Zhubin Gahvari, MD
University of Wisconsin Carbone Cancer Center

Guillermo Garcia-Manero, MD
The University of Texas MD Anderson Cancer Center

Aaron Goldberg, MD, PhD
Memorial Sloan Kettering Cancer Center

*Elizabeth A. Griffiths, MD
Roswell Park Comprehensive Cancer Center

Tamanna Haque, MD
Memorial Sloan Kettering Cancer Center

Meagan Jacoby, MD, PhD
Siteman Cancer Center at Barnes-Jewish Hospital and Washington University School of Medicine

Brian A. Jonas, MD, PhD
UC Davis Comprehensive Cancer Center

Sioban Keel, MD
Fred Hutchinson Cancer Center

Rashmi Khanal, MD
Fox Chase Cancer Center

Ashwin Kishtagari, MD
Vanderbilt-Ingram Cancer Center

Yazan Madanat, MD
UT Southwestern Simmons Comprehensive Cancer Center

Lori J. Maness, MD
Fred & Pamela Buffett Cancer Center

Shannon McCurdy, MD
Abramson Cancer Center at the University of Pennsylvania

Christine McMahon, MD
University of Colorado Cancer Center

Olatoyosi Odenike, MD
The UChicago Medicine Comprehensive Cancer Cetner

Afaf Osman, MD
Huntsman Cancer Institute at the University of Utah

*Vishnu V. Reddy, MD
O'Neal Comprehensive Cancer Center at UAB

David A. Sallman, MD
Moffitt Cancer Center

Hamid Sayar, MD, MSc
Indiana University Melvin and Bren Simon Comprehensive Cancer Center

Rory Shallis, MD
Yale Cancer Center/Smilow Cancer Hospital

Abhay Singh, MD, MPH
Case Comprehensive Cancer Center/ University Hospitals Seidman Cancer Center and Cleveland Clinic Taussig Cancer Institute

Tiffany Tanaka, MD
UC San Diego Moores Cancer Center

Swapna Thota, MD
St. Jude Children's Research Hospital/ The University of Tennessee Health Science Center

NCCN

Carly Cassara, MSc
Guidelines Layout Specialist

Mary Dwyer, MS
Senior Director, Guidelines Operations

Cindy Hochstetler, PhD
Oncology Scientist/Senior Medical Writer

Emily Kovach
Guidelines Layout Specialist

* Reviewed this patient guide. For disclosures, visit NCCN.org/disclosures.

NCCN Cancer Centers

Abramson Cancer Center
at the University of Pennsylvania
Philadelphia, Pennsylvania
800.789.7366 • pennmedicine.org/cancer

Case Comprehensive Cancer Center/
University Hospitals Seidman Cancer Center and
Cleveland Clinic Taussig Cancer Institute
Cleveland, Ohio
UH Seidman Cancer Center
800.641.2422 • uhhospitals.org/services/cancer-services
CC Taussig Cancer Institute
866.223.8100 • my.clevelandclinic.org/departments/cancer
Case CCC
216.844.8797 • case.edu/cancer

City of Hope National Medical Center
Duarte, California
800.826.4673 • cityofhope.org

Dana-Farber/Brigham and Women's Cancer Center |
Mass General Cancer Center
Boston, Massachusetts
877.442.3324 • youhaveus.org
617.726.5130 • massgeneral.org/cancer-center

Duke Cancer Institute
Durham, North Carolina
888.275.3853 • dukecancerinstitute.org

Fox Chase Cancer Center
Philadelphia, Pennsylvania
888.369.2427 • foxchase.org

Fred & Pamela Buffett Cancer Center
Omaha, Nebraska
402.559.5600 • unmc.edu/cancercenter

Fred Hutchinson Cancer Center
Seattle, Washington
206.667.5000 • fredhutch.org

Huntsman Cancer Institute at the University of Utah
Salt Lake City, Utah
800.824.2073 • healthcare.utah.edu/huntsmancancerinstitute

Indiana University Melvin and Bren Simon
Comprehensive Cancer Center
Indianapolis, Indiana
888.600.4822 • www.cancer.iu.edu

Johns Hopkins Kimmel Cancer Center
Baltimore, Maryland
410.955.8964
www.hopkinskimmelcancercenter.org

Mayo Clinic Comprehensive Cancer Center
Phoenix/Scottsdale, Arizona
Jacksonville, Florida
Rochester, Minnesota
480.301.8000 • Arizona
904.953.0853 • Florida
507.538.3270 • Minnesota
mayoclinic.org/cancercenter

Memorial Sloan Kettering Cancer Center
New York, New York
800.525.2225 • mskcc.org

Moffitt Cancer Center
Tampa, Florida
888.663.3488 • moffitt.org

O'Neal Comprehensive Cancer Center at UAB
Birmingham, Alabama
800.822.0933 • uab.edu/onealcancercenter

Robert H. Lurie Comprehensive Cancer Center
of Northwestern University
Chicago, Illinois
866.587.4322 • cancer.northwestern.edu

Roswell Park Comprehensive Cancer Center
Buffalo, New York
877.275.7724 • roswellpark.org

Siteman Cancer Center at Barnes-Jewish Hospital
and Washington University School of Medicine
St. Louis, Missouri
800.600.3606 • siteman.wustl.edu

St. Jude Children's Research Hospital/
The University of Tennessee Health Science Center
Memphis, Tennessee
866.278.5833 • stjude.org
901.448.5500 • uthsc.edu

Stanford Cancer Institute
Stanford, California
877.668.7535 • cancer.stanford.edu

The Ohio State University Comprehensive Cancer Center -
James Cancer Hospital and Solove Research Institute
Columbus, Ohio
800.293.5066 • cancer.osu.edu

The UChicago Medicine Comprehensive Cancer Center
Chicago, Illinois
773.702.1000 • uchicagomedicine.org/cancer

The University of Texas MD Anderson Cancer Center
Houston, Texas
844.269.5922 • mdanderson.org

UC Davis Comprehensive Cancer Center
Sacramento, California
916.734.5959 • 800.770.9261
health.ucdavis.edu/cancer

UC San Diego Moores Cancer Center
La Jolla, California
858.822.6100 • cancer.ucsd.edu

UCLA Jonsson Comprehensive Cancer Center
Los Angeles, California
310.825.5268 • uclahealth.org/cancer

UCSF Helen Diller Family
Comprehensive Cancer Center
San Francisco, California
800.689.8273 • cancer.ucsf.edu

University of Colorado Cancer Center
Aurora, Colorado
720.848.0300 • coloradocancercenter.org

University of Michigan Rogel Cancer Center
Ann Arbor, Michigan
800.865.1125 • rogelcancercenter.org

University of Wisconsin Carbone Cancer Center
Madison, Wisconsin
608.265.1700 • uwhealth.org/cancer

UT Southwestern Simmons
Comprehensive Cancer Center
Dallas, Texas
214.648.3111 • utsouthwestern.edu/simmons

Vanderbilt-Ingram Cancer Center
Nashville, Tennessee
877.936.8422 • vicc.org

Yale Cancer Center/Smilow Cancer Hospital
New Haven, Connecticut
855.4.SMILOW • yalecancercenter.org

share with us.

Take our survey and help make the NCCN Guidelines for Patients better for everyone!

NCCN.org/patients/comments

Notes

Index

Made in the USA
Coppell, TX
20 September 2025

60267355R00043